COMPLETE GUIDE TO HERNIA REPAIR SURGERY

Comprehensive Handbook To Procedures, Recovery, And Minimizing Complications For Effective Treatment

DR. BRUNO HORAN

Copyright © 2023 by Dr. Bruno Horan

All rights reserved. Except for brief quotations embodied in critical reviews and certain other noncommercial uses permitted by copyright law, no part of this publication may be reproduced, distributed, or transmitted in any form or by any means, Including photocopying, recording, or other electronic or mechanical methods, without the prior written permission of the publisher.

Disclaimer:

The information provided in this book, is intended for general informational purposes only and should not be considered as professional advice.

The author has made every effort to ensure the accuracy of the information presented. However, readers are advised to consult with a qualified healthcare professional before attempting any herbal remedies or making significant changes to their wellness routine. Individual health conditions vary, and what may be suitable for one person may not be appropriate for another.

It is important to note that the author is not in any endorsement deal, partnership, or affiliation with any organization, brand, or company mentioned in this book. Any references to specific products or services are based on the author's personal experience or general knowledge and do not imply an endorsement or promotion of those products or services

Contents

CHAPTER ONE 13
  RECOGNIZING HERNIAS 13
    The Meaning And Kinds Of Hernias 13
    Reasons And Danger Elements 14
    Signs And Prognosis 15
    The Value Of Prompt Intervention 16
    An Overview Of Available Therapies 17

CHAPTER TWO 19
  GETTING READY FOR SURGERY 19
    Pre-Operative Evaluations 19
    Selecting A Suitable Surgeon 20
    Pre-Optional Lifestyle Modifications 22
    Recognizing Your Surgical Options 23
    Getting Ready For The Recuperation Phase 24

CHAPTER THREE 27
  HERNIA REPAIR SURGERY OPEN 27
    Procedure Step-By-Step For Surgery 27
    Taking Care Of The Hernia Defect: 28
    Timeline For Recuperation 30
    Patient Outcomes And Success Rates 33

CHAPTER FOUR 35
SURGERY FOR LAPAROSCOPIC HERNIA REPAIR ... 35
Procedure Step-By-Step For Surgery 35
Positives And Negatives 37
Timeline For Recuperation 38
Possible Difficulties 40
Patient Outcomes And Success Rates 41
CHAPTER FIVE 43
AFTER SURGERY CARE 43
Quick Post-Operative Treatment 43
Techniques For Pain Management 44
Gradual Resumption Of Regular Activities 45
Keeping An Eye Out For Complications 46
Expectations For A Long-Term Recovery 47
CHAPTER SIX 49
TAKING CARE OF COMPLEXITIES 49
Typical Post-Op Complications 49
Early Warning Indications 49
Options For Complication Treatment 50
Preventive Actions 50

When To Get Medical Assistance 51
CHAPTER SEVEN 53
　ADVANCES IN LIFESTYLE POST-SURGERY 53
　　Tips For Nutrition And Diet 53
　　Guidelines For Physical Activity And Exercise 54
　　Steer Clear Of Strain And Injury 55
　　Extended Lifestyle Adjustments 56
　　Sustaining General Health 57
CHAPTER EIGHT 59
　TRIBUTES AND TESTIMONIALS FROM PATIENTS .. 59
　　Actual Experiences 59
　　Advice From Former Patients 60
　　Overcoming Obstacles 62
　　Motivation And Encouragement 64

CONCERNING THIS BOOK

"Hernia Repair Surgery" is a thorough manual created to provide patients with the information they need to successfully navigate the challenging hernia treatment process.

This book starts off by giving readers a basic grasp of hernias, including information on their many forms, underlying causes, and risk factors. Hernias are a prevalent condition that is sometimes misinterpreted. Readers who are able to identify the symptoms and comprehend the diagnostic procedure will be better able to seek prompt medical assistance, which is essential for avoiding complications and guaranteeing the best possible results.

The book examines the variety of treatment methods available and stresses the significance of early intervention.

It walks patients through the pre-operative period, emphasizing the value of comprehensive pre-operative evaluations, choosing a qualified surgeon, and implementing the required lifestyle changes. The book intends to reduce fear and promote informed decision-making by demystifying surgery and preparing people for recovery.

The book provides thorough, step-by-step explanations of each operation in the sections devoted to open hernia surgery, laparoscopic hernia repair, and robotic-assisted hernia repair. Patients can choose their treatments wisely by weighing the advantages, disadvantages, recovery times, and any consequences.

This comprehensive analysis gives a realistic picture of what to expect by including success rates and patient outcomes as well.

A good recovery after surgery depends on post-operative care, and this book provides thorough instructions on pain management, returning to normal activities, and keeping an eye out for problems.

It offers helpful guidance on long-term rehabilitation, stressing the value of ongoing monitoring and follow-up care.

The book also covers another important topic, which is handling problems. Through providing them with knowledge about frequent post-surgery problems, early warning signals, and available therapies, patients are empowered to take charge of their own recovery. In order to ensure that readers are ready for everything, the book also discusses preventive measures and offers advice on when to seek medical attention.

Following surgery, changing one's lifestyle is essential for preserving health and avoiding recurrence. The book provides helpful advice on physical activity, diet, nutrition, and exercise as well as ways to prevent strain and injury. It supports long-term lifestyle modifications that help patients maintain their general well-being.

A personal touch is added by including patient stories and testimonials, which provide advice, encouragement, and real-life experiences from people who have successfully overcome the difficulties associated with hernia repair surgery. These stories inspire and reassure readers, making them feel understood and supported all along the way.

CHAPTER ONE

RECOGNIZING HERNIAS

The Meaning And Kinds Of Hernias

An internal organ or tissue that protrudes through a weak area in the muscle or tissue that should hold it in place results in a hernia. Hernias come in a variety of forms, each called for the area in which they develop:

The most prevalent kind of hernia is inguinal; it develops in the groin, where the thigh and abdomen meet.

Femoral Hernia: Found closer to the thigh and situated lower down than inguinal hernias.

Found close to the navel or belly button, umbilical hernias are frequently observed in newborns.

An incisional hernia is a growth that occurs where a prior surgical incision is made.

A hiatal hernia occurs when the upper stomach pushes into the chest cavity through the diaphragm.

The severity of each form of hernia might vary, and they may also provide unique treatment and symptom issues.

Reasons And Danger Elements

Generally, a combination of strain and muscle weakness results in the development of hernias. Hernias can result from the following factors:

Experiencing strain when performing strenuous physical work or heavy lifting.

Chronic Coughing: Recurrent coughing caused by illnesses such as chronic obstructive pulmonary disease (COPD).

Pregnancy: Umbilical hernias, in particular, can develop as a result of abdominal strain.

Obesity: Carrying too much weight increases the risk of hernias and weakens the abdominal muscles.

Age: Aging can cause muscle weakening and connective tissue degradation, which makes older persons more vulnerable.

Signs And Prognosis

Depending on the kind and location, a hernia's symptoms might vary but often include:

Visible Lump: Usually the initial symptom, particularly while standing or exerting oneself.

Pain or Unease: Particularly when coughing, bending over, or lifting.

A burning or hurting feeling, especially where the lump is.

A sensation of fullness in the lower abdomen or groin.

A physical examination is usually required for diagnosis. During this procedure, the doctor will feel for any lumps and may ask you to cough or strain in order to check for any more hernia protrusions.

For confirmation, imaging tests like an MRI or ultrasound may be performed, particularly if the hernia is difficult to feel.

The Value Of Prompt Intervention

In order to avoid problems like incarceration or strangulation, where the projecting tissue becomes trapped and its blood supply is cut off, timely treatment of hernias is essential.

Serious discomfort, tissue damage, and in rare instances, potentially fatal conditions necessitating immediate surgery can result from these complications.

An Overview Of Available Therapies

The kind, size, symptoms, and general health of the patient are some of the aspects that determine the available treatment choices for hernias. Treatment typically falls into one of two categories:

Non-Surgical Handling:

When a small hernia is not producing severe symptoms, it can be treated as follows:

Be vigilant in keeping an eye out for any changes or symptoms related to the hernia.

Use of Trusses or Belts: These devices, which can support a hernia, are less frequently advised these days because of the possible risks.

Surgical Restoration:

Surgery is usually necessary for most hernias in order to fortify the weak spot and close the abdominal wall aperture. Typical surgical methods include:

Open Surgery: A conventional technique in which the surgeon creates a cut close to the hernia location and repairs the deformity with synthetic mesh or sutures.

Laparoscopic Surgery: This minimally invasive procedure uses specialized devices and a camera to fix a hernia through a series of tiny incisions. Compared to open surgery, this method usually causes less discomfort and requires a shorter recovery period.

CHAPTER TWO

GETTING READY FOR SURGERY

Pre-Operative Evaluations

To make sure you are safe and prepared for the procedure, a number of pre-operative evaluations are usually carried out before hernia repair surgery.

A physical examination, blood tests, and even imaging procedures like an ultrasound or CT scan are some of the possible components of these evaluations.

The goal is to assess your general state of health, locate any underlying medical issues that may impact surgery, and choose the best course of action for your particular situation.

Your doctor will measure the hernia's size and location during the physical examination and look for any indications of potential consequences including strangling, which occurs when the herniated tissue's blood supply is cut off. Blood tests provide vital information for surgery planning by assessing your blood count, renal function, and electrolyte levels. When making surgical decisions, imaging tests can help by providing precise views of the hernia and adjacent structures.

In order to customize the surgical approach to your specific needs and guarantee the surgery is as safe and effective as possible, these assessments are crucial.

They also give your medical staff the opportunity to address any worries you may have by going over any possible risks or consequences with you in advance.

Selecting A Suitable Surgeon

One of the most important choices you will have to make when getting ready for hernia repair surgery is choosing a skilled specialist. A competent surgeon has to be board-certified, possess a great deal of expertise performing hernia procedures, and ideally specialize in the particular kind of hernia you have.

You can look up possible surgeons online, get referrals from friends who have had comparable operations done or your primary care physician, and arrange meetings to talk about your case.

Make sure to enquire about the surgeon's success rate, experience, and any possible side effects throughout your appointment regarding hernia repairs.

Prior to having surgery, it is critical that you have complete trust and confidence in your surgeon. A skilled surgeon will also take the time to address any concerns you may have about the surgery and to go over the surgical strategy they prescribe for you.

Pre-Optional Lifestyle Modifications

Prior to hernia repair surgery, a few lifestyle changes might assist maximize your recovery and overall results.

To reduce the dangers associated with surgery, your surgeon may advise you to refrain from smoking and to drink less alcohol in addition to keeping a nutritious diet that will aid in recovering.

It's critical to properly manage any chronic medical illnesses, such as diabetes or hypertension, prior to surgery in order to minimize complications.

By maintaining your level of physical activity, you can enhance your recuperation by increasing your muscle tone and circulation.

Exercises or other activities tailored to strengthening abdominal muscles may be recommended by your surgeon to help with your rehabilitation following surgery. A more seamless recovery process can also be achieved by setting up your home to be accessible and comfortable during the healing phase.

Recognizing Your Surgical Options

Knowing the many surgical procedures available for hernia repair will help you and your physician make an educated decision. Open hernia repair and laparoscopic hernia repair are the two main methods. In an open hernia repair, the abdominal wall is strengthened by the surgeon using mesh patches or stitches to press the protruding tissue back into place. This procedure entails creating an incision directly over the hernia.

Known as minimally invasive surgery, laparoscopic hernia repair entails making multiple tiny incisions to introduce a camera and surgical equipment. Using magnified images on a monitor, the surgeon guides the mending procedure with the help of the camera. Compared to open surgery, this method typically produces fewer scars, less pain after surgery, and a quicker recovery.

Depending on the location and extent of the hernia, your general health, and your preferences, your surgeon will advise you on the best course of action. They will walk you through the advantages and possible drawbacks of each method so you can take an active part in choosing which one to use.

Getting Ready For The Recuperation Phase

A smooth recovery following hernia repair surgery can be ensured by taking a few practical steps in advance of the recovery period. recommendations pertaining to your case will be given by your surgeon, but in general, you should prepare for enough rest and take time off work or other normal activities as needed. Having basic materials on hand, such as painkillers, bandages, and quick-to-prepare foods, will make your recuperation at home easier.

It can also be helpful to make arrangements for family or friends to aid you in the early postoperative days, particularly if you anticipate needing assistance with everyday duties or transportation. You will be able to schedule follow-up consultations with your surgeon to discuss any concerns you may have during the recovery time and to track your healing progress.

You can improve your chances of a successful outcome and your experience with hernia repair surgery by adhering to these suggestions and preparations. To effectively support your recovery process, remember to ask questions, be open with your medical staff, and follow their advice.

CHAPTER THREE

HERNIA REPAIR SURGERY OPEN

A popular treatment used to treat a hernia is hernia repair surgery. A hernia is a condition in which an internal organ or tissue protrudes through a weak point in the surrounding muscle or connective tissue. The purpose of the procedure is to strengthen the weak spot and relieve hernia-related discomfort.

Procedure Step-By-Step For Surgery

Preoperative Preparation: The medical staff will get you ready before the procedure starts. Usually, this entails giving you anesthesia so that the surgery would be painless and comfortable for you. Depending on your health status and the particular procedure you have scheduled, different types of anesthesia may be used.

Making an Incision and Getting to the Hernia: The surgeon will make an incision close to the hernia site while you are sedated. The herniated tissue or organ is accessible through this incision. Depending on the kind and location of the hernia, the incision's size and position may change.

Reduction of Herniated Tissue: The following action entails gently moving the organ or tissue that is protruding back into the abdomen or other affected location in the proper place. Reduction is the procedure that is necessary to repair the hernia.

Taking Care Of The Hernia Defect:

The surgeon will repair the weakened or damaged muscle or connective tissue that allowed the hernia to develop after decreasing the hernia. In order to give extra support and stop the hernia from happening again, this surgery is frequently completed with surgical mesh or stitches.

Closure of Incision: After the repair is finished, the surgeon will use surgical glue, staples, or stitches to close the incision. The surgeon's preference and the size of the incision determine the sort of closure method to be employed.

Positives and Negatives

Advantages:

Effective Resolution: By minimizing discomfort and averting potential problems, hernia repair surgery efficiently treats the hernia.

Better Quality of Life: Patients frequently report feeling less pain, discomfort, and bulging related to hernias.

Low Recurrence Rates: The use of mesh in modern surgery has helped to reduce the recurrence rates of hernias.

Cons:

Surgical Risks: Following any operation, there is a chance of developing complications like bleeding, infection, or anesthesia-related side effects.

Recuperation Time: Following hernia repair surgery, recovery times might differ. Some patients may feel uncomfortable or find it difficult to engage in certain physical activities while they heal.

Cost: The cost of hernia repair surgery varies depending on the type of procedure and insurance coverage.

Timeline For Recuperation

Following hernia repair surgery, recovery times can vary based on a number of variables, including the type of operation and the patient's health. Typically, patients should anticipate:

Immediate Postoperative Period: Following surgery, you will be monitored by a doctor as you recover in the recovery area.

During this stage, the management of pain and the observation of any emerging problems are of utmost importance.

First Few Days: In the vicinity of the surgery site, you can feel sore, swollen, and have limited mobility. Adherence to postoperative care recommendations for wound care, medication administration, and activity limitations is imperative.

First Few Weeks: Your strength and mobility will gradually return. Most patients can return to work and light activities in a few weeks, but you should avoid doing anything too rigorous until your surgeon gives the all-clear.

Long-Term Recovery: Following hernia repair surgery, you should schedule follow-up consultations with your healthcare practitioner to check healing and address any issues.

Full recovery from this type of surgery typically takes several weeks to months.

Possible Difficulties

Although hernia repair surgery is usually safe, the following side effects could occur:

Infection at the Surgical Site: To reduce the risk of infection, proper wound care and hygiene are essential.

Hematoma or Excessive Bleeding: In rare circumstances, a hematoma—a collection of blood—may form close to the surgery site.

Nerve Damage: Numbness, tingling, or weakness may result from transient or, in rare cases, chronic nerve damage close to the surgery site.

Hernia Recurrence: Even with improvements in surgical methods, hernias can sometimes reoccur and require additional care.

Patient Outcomes And Success Rates

Hernia repair surgery has a high success rate overall, with many patients reporting significant symptom reduction and long-term hernia resolution.

Success depends on the kind of hernia, the surgical method, and the patient's health. Typical patient outcomes include:

Pain, discomfort, and swelling are among the symptoms that patients usually report being relieved.

Low Recurrence Rates: The chance of a hernia recurrence has decreased because of modern procedures such as mesh repairs that don't require tension.

Better Quality of Life: After a successful surgical procedure, patients can frequently return to their regular activities without the restrictions a hernia imposes.

You may better prepare for hernia repair surgery and make healthcare decisions if you are aware of the technique, recovery time, and possible results.

CHAPTER FOUR

SURGERY FOR LAPAROSCOPIC HERNIA REPAIR

Procedure Step-By-Step For Surgery

General anesthesia is given before laparoscopic hernia repair surgery to guarantee that the patient is totally unconscious and pain-free for the entire process. The surgeon makes a few tiny abdominal incisions after the patient is sedated.

The laparoscope and surgical equipment are inserted through these incisions, which are usually smaller than an inch in length.

Through one of the incisions, the laparoscope—a narrow tube with a high-definition camera and light—is introduced.

The surgeon may observe the hernia and surrounding tissues in excellent detail thanks to the camera's real-time image transmission to a monitor. With this minimally invasive method, a major incision is not necessary to get a clear picture.

Through the remaining wounds, the physician then inserts specialty surgical equipment. Using these tools, the protruding tissue or organ is gently pushed back into position.

A synthetic mesh is placed over the weak spot after the hernia has been minimized. By strengthening the abdominal wall, this mesh stops the hernia from happening again. Tissue glue, staples, or sutures are typically used to hold the mesh in place.

The surgeon gently removes the laparoscope and instruments after making sure the mesh is positioned and secured appropriately.

Sutures or surgical glue are then used to seal the tiny incisions. Ultimately, a sterile bandage is used to shield the cuts and encourage their healing.

Depending on how complicated the hernia is, the complete process usually takes one to two hours.

Positives And Negatives

Compared to open surgery, laparoscopic hernia repair surgery has a number of advantages. The procedure's least invasiveness is one of its biggest advantages. Less pain and recovery time are experienced after laparoscopic surgery because of the small incisions made during the procedure. After a few weeks, patients can usually resume their regular activities, but open surgery takes many months.

Laparoscopic surgery also lowers the risk of complications and infection. Reduced exposure to external pollutants due to smaller incisions lowers the risk of wound infections.

Better long-term results may result from more accurate repairs made possible by the laparoscope's comprehensive vision.

Laparoscopic hernia repair is not without its problems, though. Not all medical facilities may have the particular expertise and experience needed for the surgery.

Additionally, general anesthesia is used, which entails risks of its own, especially for patients with underlying medical issues. In certain instances, if complications develop or if the hernia is too complicated to fix laparoscopically, the surgeon might have to switch to an open operation.

Timeline For Recuperation

Compared to open surgery, laparoscopic hernia repair surgery typically has a faster recovery period and less pain.

The majority of patients can typically return home the same day or the day following their surgery. Managing the pain and suffering during the initial stages of recuperation is usually easy and can be accomplished with over-the-counter pain medicines.

Patients are instructed to rest and refrain from heavy activity during the first week following surgery. It is advised to take short walks to enhance blood flow and avoid blood clots.

Depending on their line of work, many patients can resume light activities and go back to work by the second week.

Four to six weeks is usually enough time for full recovery, which includes resumed exercise and all other regular activities.

To ensure proper healing of the abdominal wall, patients are advised to refrain from heavy lifting and strenuous exercise during this period.

The surgeon will schedule follow-up appointments to monitor the healing process and address any concerns.

Possible Difficulties

Complications are possible with laparoscopic hernia repair surgery, just like with any surgical procedure. These may include bleeding, anesthesia-related side effects, and infection at the site of the incisions. In certain cases, nerve irritation or the body's reaction to the mesh may be the cause of persistent pain or discomfort in the repaired area for some patients.

Other potential complications include hernia recurrence, which may occur if the repair is not sufficiently reinforced or if the patient engages in strenuous activities too soon after surgery. In rare circumstances, the mesh can move or create an inflammatory reaction, prompting additional surgery to treat these difficulties.

More significant but infrequent problems include injury to nearby organs, such as the intestines or bladder, during the treatment. The surgeon's experience and the use of cutting-edge imaging methods reduce this danger. Any unexpected symptoms, such as intense pain, fever, or infection-related symptoms, should be reported by patients to their healthcare physician right once.

Patient Outcomes And Success Rates

The majority of research shows that laparoscopic hernia repair surgery has a high success rate of over 90%. Because it is less intrusive and has a decreased risk of complications, this procedure has become the recommended option for hernia repair.

Patient outcomes are generally excellent, with many finding great alleviation from symptoms and a low probability of hernia recurrence.

Long-term outcomes are equally positive, with the majority of patients returning to their typical activities without further difficulties. The use of synthetic mesh has been shown to offer robust and lasting support to the healed area, lowering the likelihood of future hernias. However, individual outcomes can vary based on factors such as the patient's overall health, the size and location of the hernia, and adherence to postoperative care guidelines.

Patients are recommended to follow their surgeon's advice closely, including attending follow-up consultations and following activity limits during the recovery period.

Proper postoperative care and lifestyle adjustments, such as keeping a healthy weight and avoiding hard lifting, can further enhance the success and longevity of the hernia repair.

CHAPTER FIVE

AFTER SURGERY CARE

Quick Post-Operative Treatment

Immediate post-operative care following hernia repair surgery is essential for a successful recovery. Usually, patients are taken to a recovery room where medical staff keeps a careful eye on them.

Regular checks are made on vital signs such as blood pressure, heart rate, and oxygen saturation. Additionally, the surgical site is inspected for evidence of severe bleeding or edema.

In order to reduce strain on the surgical region, it is crucial to rest and refrain from engaging in any vigorous activity during this early phase.

Because of the anesthesia, patients may feel sleepy or confused; therefore, having a family member or friend nearby can be comforting and helpful.

Techniques For Pain Management

After hernia repair surgery, pain is a typical issue, but there are a number of effective techniques to control it.

Physicians frequently recommend over-the-counter painkillers such as acetaminophen or ibuprofen, as well as stronger prescription drugs as needed.

To further reduce swelling and numb the surgical site, ice packs can be administered. This will also help with pain relief.

It's also a good idea to approach physical exercise gradually and gently, avoiding any motions that make you uncomfortable.

Exercises that involve deep breathing and relaxation can help control pain and lower tension, which can facilitate a quicker recovery.

Gradual Resumption Of Regular Activities

Resuming regular activities ought to be done cautiously and gradually. Patients are first instructed to refrain from heavy lifting, vigorous exercise, and any other activity that puts tension on the abdominal muscles.

Soon after surgery, light exercises like walking can be resumed to improve circulation and avoid blood clots. Patients can gradually resume more activity as their healing advances, but it's important to pay attention to their bodies and refrain from overexerting themselves.

Schedule follow-up consultations with the surgeon to monitor the healing process and assess whether it's safe to resume strenuous activities such as work and exercise.

Keeping An Eye Out For Complications

One of the most important aspects of postoperative treatment is keeping an eye out for any problems. Increased redness, swelling, or discharge from the surgery site, together with prolonged fever, excruciating pain, or trouble urinating, are typical indicators of problems.

Reporting any of these symptoms to a healthcare professional right away is advised. Complications like infections or hernia recurrences might happen occasionally and need for immediate medical intervention.

Frequent follow-up appointments with the surgeon reduce the chance of long-term complications by ensuring that any difficulties are identified and treated promptly.

Expectations For A Long-Term Recovery

The type of hernia and the particular surgical technique used to determine the length of recuperation following hernia repair surgery.

Within a few weeks to a few months, the majority of patients can anticipate a progressive improvement in their symptoms and a return to their regular activities.

Maintaining a healthy lifestyle, which includes eating a balanced diet and getting regular exercise, is crucial to promoting healing and preventing recurrence.

Additionally, patients should adhere to any special advice given by their medical team, such as wearing supportive clothing or refraining from heavy lifting for a predetermined amount of time.

Most people who receive the right care and attention after surgery can recover completely and have an improved quality of life.

CHAPTER SIX

TAKING CARE OF COMPLEXITIES

Typical Post-Op Complications

Despite the success of the treatment, some individuals may have difficulties following hernia repair surgery. Infection is a common consequence that shows up at the surgery site as redness, swelling, or discharge. Recurrence of the hernia is another problem, in which the repaired tissue weakens or tears once more, resulting in discomfort or a discernible bulge. Because of muscle strain or irritation of the nerves throughout the healing process, pain and discomfort around the surgical site may not go away.

Early Warning Indications

Early detection of surgical complications is essential for timely treatment. Keep an eye out for signs like fever, chills, swelling that becomes worse over time, or increased pain that doesn't go away when you take painkillers. Indications that need medical care include extensive drainage or pus, redness, and warmth surrounding the surgical site.

Options For Complication Treatment

Depending on the particular problem, several treatments are used for post-surgery problems. Antibiotics are usually used to cure infections, although further surgery to reinforce the weak area may be necessary in cases with recurrent hernias. Medication or physical therapy are two examples of pain management techniques that can be used to treat chronic pain or nerve-related problems.

Preventive Actions

Following hernia repair surgery, a number of precautions can assist avoid problems. Risks can be reduced by closely adhering to post-operative care recommendations, which include keeping the surgical site dry and clean, avoiding physically demanding activities, and wearing supportive clothing as directed by your surgeon. Remaining smoke-free and maintaining a healthy weight also improve surgery outcomes and lower the risk of complications.

When To Get Medical Assistance

Knowing when to seek emergency medical attention following hernia repair surgery is crucial. Get in touch with your healthcare provider right once if you have extreme pain that doesn't go away despite taking recommended medicine, unexpected swelling or redness that extends beyond the surgery site, fever, or ongoing nausea and vomiting. Prompt action helps ensure a smooth healing process and stop issues from getting worse.

CHAPTER SEVEN

ADVANCES IN LIFESTYLE POST-SURGERY

Tips For Nutrition And Diet

A healthy, well-balanced diet is essential to your recuperation following hernia repair surgery. To avoid putting undue strain on your abdominal muscles, your food should start out light and simple to digest. Start with clear liquids, such as broths, then work your way up to soft foods, like yogurt, applesauce, and oats. Focus on including high-fiber foods in your regular diet as you make the switch from a restricted one to avoid constipation, which can put a strain on your surgery site. Whole grains, legumes, fruits, and veggies are all great options.

Incorporate lean meats, fish, eggs, beans, and nuts into your diet as they are high in protein and necessary for tissue repair. Drink lots of water throughout the day to stay hydrated. Foods that produce gas or bloating should be avoided as well as carbonated beverages, as they might raise abdominal pressure. Limiting alcohol and caffeine during the early stages of recovery is also a good idea because they can dehydrate you and impede healing.

Guidelines For Physical Activity And Exercise

Exercise is crucial to the healing process, but it must be done carefully. Focus on light movement in the initial days following surgery to encourage blood flow without straining the surgical site. Frequent short walks can help avoid blood clots and improve overall healing.

Gradually up the duration and intensity of your workouts as you recover. Until your doctor provides the all-clear, refrain from heavy lifting, strenuous exercise, and any other activity that puts undue strain on your abdominal muscles for at least six weeks.

When you resume your exercise regimen, choose low-impact sports like cycling, walking, or swimming. Always pay attention to your body's signals and cease any action that hurts or creates discomfort.

Steer Clear Of Strain And Injury

It is essential to refrain from activities that put tension on your abdominal area in order to avoid complications and guarantee a speedy recovery.

This includes coughing up a lot, lifting big things, and doing intense physical activity. Use the right form when lifting something: bend your knees, maintain a straight back, and lift with your leg muscles.

Steer clear of sitting or standing still for extended periods of time. Take pauses to stretch and walk about. Use your hand or a small pillow to support your incision whenever you need to cough or sneeze in order to lessen the pressure.

Additionally, avoiding constipation is crucial because straining during bowel movements might impede your recovery. To combat constipation, eat a high-fiber diet and stay hydrated.

Extended Lifestyle Adjustments

Making long-term lifestyle adjustments can improve your general health and help you avoid hernias in the future. Keep your weight within a healthy range; too much weight puts strain on your abdominal muscles and increases your risk of hernias. It's important to exercise regularly but concentrate on core-strengthening activities that won't strain your muscles.

If you haven't already, give up smoking since it might hinder tissue recovery and raise the possibility of problems.

Additionally, take care of any allergies or a persistent cough that can lead to frequent coughing, which can put a strain on your abdominal muscles.

It's critical to pay attention to your body's cues and to seek medical attention if you experience any strange symptoms.

Sustaining General Health

Taking a holistic approach to health will help you heal and avoid hernias in the future. Make sure you get adequate sleep because recovery and general well-being depend on slumber. Use stress-reduction methods including yoga, meditation, and deep breathing. Stress can impair your immune system and make recovery more difficult.

It's crucial to schedule routine check-ups with your healthcare practitioner to track your progress and quickly treat any issues. Following these recommendations and leading a conscientious lifestyle can help you recuperate from hernia repair surgery and preserve your long-term health.

CHAPTER EIGHT

TRIBUTES AND TESTIMONIALS FROM PATIENTS

Actual Experiences

Patients' first-hand accounts of their hernia repair surgeries offer priceless insights into what to anticipate during the process.

Many patients remember their feelings of worry leading up to surgery because they had no idea what to expect. John, a 45-year-old engineer, for instance, described how he found out he had a hernia during a standard check-up.

He was a little uncomfortable at first, but it got worse with time. He made the decision to consult a doctor, who suggested surgery. John talked about how the medical staff allayed his anxieties by thoroughly explaining the operation. Despite occasional challenges, his post-surgery rehabilitation was effectively managed with appropriate direction and assistance, enabling him to fully resume his active lifestyle.

Maria, a 35-year-old teacher who was one of the patients, described her experience with an umbilical hernia. Her experience demonstrated the value of prompt diagnosis and care. Maria became aware of a tiny bulge close to her navel and made the quick decision to consult a doctor. After making a snap choice, she underwent a minimally invasive laparoscopic procedure, and in a few weeks, she was back to her regular activities. Maria stressed how relieved she was to have taken care of the problem before it became worse.

Advice From Former Patients

Patients who have undergone hernia repair surgery frequently offer insightful counsel to those who will be undergoing the operation. One popular piece of advice is to plan ahead for the recuperation phase. This entails creating a cozy area at home with all the necessities—like pillows, entertainment, and basic supplies—within easy reach. Alice, a sixty-year-old retiree, advised making plans for assistance in the early days following surgery. She discovered that having her daughter stay with her during the first week helped her recuperate considerably.

Dietary modifications are also very important. A high-fiber diet is advised by many patients in order to avoid constipation, which can be a typical side effect of painkillers following surgery. The healing process can be considerably sped up by drinking plenty of water and adhering to the surgeon's dietary recommendations. Reintroducing physical activity should be done gradually. Past patients emphasize the value of following the medical team's advice to move gently and refrain from heavy lifting until completely healed.

Overcoming Obstacles

Hernia repair surgery recovery has a unique set of obstacles, but it can be tremendously uplifting to see how others have surmounted them. The most difficult thing to do is manage pain and discomfort. It's important for patients to adhere to the recommended pain management plan, which may include taking medications and getting enough rest. Other techniques, such as using ice packs and giving the surgery site a light massage, have helped some people find relief.

Emotional obstacles may also surface, such as annoyance at the momentary loss of autonomy or a slower-than-anticipated rate of recuperation. Mary, a fifty-year-old administrative assistant, talked about how difficult it was for her to be patient while she healed. She took comfort in daily goal-setting that was manageable and in commemorating her accomplishments. Her surgeon's follow-up visits on a regular basis also gave her confidence and helped her stay on course.

Achievements

There are many hernia repair surgery success tales, which give encouragement to individuals who are about to have the surgery. The 30-year-old athlete David's athletic career was in jeopardy due to an inguinal hernia. After the procedure, he was able to resume his training regimen and even set new personal records thanks to a well-organized recovery program. His tale serves as evidence of both the body's amazing capacity for healing and the efficacy of contemporary surgical methods.

The inspirational recovery tale of 42-year-old Sarah, a mother of two, who battled a recurring hernia, is another. She underwent a more involved surgical repair, and through focused physical therapy, she not only totally healed but also gained new power in her core muscles. Her story emphasizes the value of tenacity and the assistance of professionals in attaining a full recovery.

Motivation And Encouragement

Although having hernia repair surgery can be frightening, previous patients' support and inspiration can be quite helpful. Numerous patients highlight the benefits and the ability to lead pain-free lives again. For example, Mark, a 55-year-old musician, explained how his performance had been hampered by his hernia. After the procedure, he was pain-free when playing his instruments, which motivated others with comparable circumstances to act.

It's critical to maintain motivation when recovering. Having reasonable objectives and savoring each tiny accomplishment will help lift spirits. Patients frequently advise joining an online or in-person support group where they may talk to people who have been through similar experiences and exchange stories. It can be energizing to know that others have made it through the healing process and that they are optimistic and dedicated to the process.

www.ingramcontent.com/pod-product-compliance
Lightning Source LLC
Chambersburg PA
CBHW071843210526
45479CB00001B/269